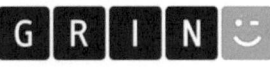

Anja Hellmann

International Migration of Nurses

Exemplary shown on the United Kingdom

GRIN Publishing

Imprint:

Copyright © 2010 GRIN Verlag, Open Publishing GmbH
Print and binding: Books on Demand GmbH, Norderstedt Germany
ISBN: 978-3-640-74914-0

This book at GRIN:

http://www.grin.com/en/e-book/158859/international-migration-of-nurses

GRIN - Your knowledge has value

Since its foundation in 1998, GRIN has specialized in publishing academic texts by students, college teachers and other academics as e-book and printed book. The website www.grin.com is an ideal platform for presenting term papers, final papers, scientific essays, dissertations and specialist books.

Visit us on the internet:

http://www.grin.com/

http://www.facebook.com/grincom

http://www.twitter.com/grin_com

International Migration of Nurses: Exemplary shown on the United Kingdom

Student: Anja Hellmann

University of Southern Denmark

Campus Esbjerg

Public Health Master

Course: Harmonization, Sovereignty, Diversity and Global Health

Content

Introduction

Migration of employees –and in particular of nurses- is no new concern. But especially the immigration from oversea nurses to the United Kingdom (UK) is highly discussed (Stilwell, 2004). Extreme nurse shortages in the UK, due to bad payment and dissatisfactory work environment, are reasons for the demand, additionally to the general demographic transition in the population with increasing demand for services, but at the same time decreasing supply of professional nurse services (Buchan, 2002). This synopsis gives an overview about the topic, its problematic sites and solutions.

1 Who are the migrating nurses?

In general there are two different groups of nurses, who are coming to the UK. Either they come from the EU/ EEA (Norway, Iceland, Liechtenstein) or from outside this region. Migrants from the EU or EEA have the right to work in another member-country. They have mostly an education as a nurse or are going to be educated in the UK

People, who are coming from outside this region normally need a verification of their qualification, which differs often between the countries (Buchan, 2002). But the UK has got a special regulation, which allows it also to work without an valid nursery exam. Domestic colleagues have then the obligation to train oversea nurses (Aiken, 2004). In contrast to the EU-region, the UK is here allowed to test nurses in their English language skills and use this as an exclusion criterion. Immigrants from this region get contracts from half a year to two years as a maximum.

The number of immigrants from the EU and EEA to the UK remains constant since many years. Due to language barriers many European nurses don´t chose often to go to the UK. The amount of nurses immigrating from outside grows steadily and is more important for the UK, because 87% (2001) of all oversea nurses are from this region. The main resource countries for the UK are the Philippines, South Africa and Australia (Tab.1). Whereas the Philippines have by far the biggest amount and this is even steadily increasing. Furthermore many nurses come from India, Zimbabwe and other African states (Tab.1) (Aiken, 2004; Buchan, 2002).

Table. Major Donor and Receiving Countries of Migrating Nurses				
Receiving countries	Australia	Canada	Ireland	UK	USA
Donor countries	China	Ireland	Australia	Australia	Canada
	Germany	Philippines	Philippines	Canada	Hong Kong
	Hong Kong	UK	UK	Finland	Japan
	India		South Africa	Germany	India
	Ireland			Ghana	Mexico
	Malaysia			Ireland	Nigeria
	New Zealand			India	Philippines
	Philippines			Kenya	Puerto Rico
	South Africa			New Zealand	South Korea
	Sri Lanka			Nigeria	UK
	UK			Pakistan	Vietnam
				Philippines	
				South Africa	
				Sweden	
				USA	
				West Indies	
				Zambia	
				Zimbabwe	

Tab.1: Major Donor and Receiving Countries of Migrating Nurses (Kline, 2003, p.108)

2 Push and Pull Factors

Push-factors, which arise from the situation in donor countries and pull- factors, which draw people to destination countries, mostly appear as a combination. Kline (2003) distinguishes between three groups of push and pull factors. The educational factors, economic/ social factors and the personal safety factors. Many nurses go to improve their professional development, their working-standards or to get a secure job (educational factors). Economic and social factors are e.g. low wages, wars, deprivation or social unrest (Stilwell, 2004). Personal safety factors can be seen on the one hand as an escape to get political safety, but on the other hand also for their health. The danger to be infected with HIV or TB is much higher in many donor countries than in the UK (Kline, 2003).

4

Buchan (2004) names groups of nurses according to their push and pull factors. One group consists of nurses, which are permanent in the UK. Those have economic reasons, are career-orientated or have a migrating partner (see also Tab.2). The second group are those, who are temporary in the UK. Those do a working holiday, a study tour, are students or (mostly) contract workers. Many of the latter ones often would like to stay longer, but are not allowed to. Furthermore different factors support the migration: Reduced regulation, like the access of Visa, is one factor. Another factor is the more and more coming professional social network or institutions, which manage the migration and build contacts from oversea nurses to the UK (Stilwell, 2004).

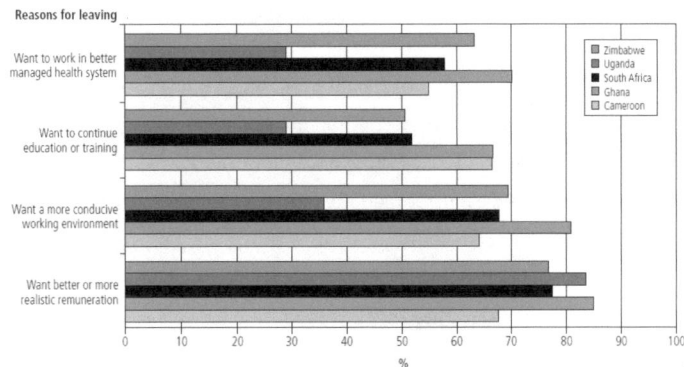

Tab.2: Factors affecting health professionals´ decision to migrate from five African countries (Stilwell, 2004, p.597)

3 Effects of migration

Two main groups are effected by migration: the countries and the migrants. For the donor countries the brain drain is the biggest negative effect. South Africa, Zimbabwe and other African states have nurse shortages and this gets even worse through the increasing emigration- mainly to the UK. A positive effect can be seen on the Philippines. Here the government supports emigration, because emigrants send their earned money to their family on the Philippines, which is then invested in the local economy. On the other side the Philippines itself gets also problems to secure the supply with nurses. But not only developing countries

5

are affected by this: The UK itself is not only a destination, but also a donor country. Due to bad working conditions and other factors many nurses go to the US, Canada and Australia (Kline, 2003). Many immigrated nurses achieve the positive effects, they wish to have in the UK. But negative effects are reported, too. Poor accommodations, undervaluing of skills, poor information about contracts, low wages and racism are the most mentioned ones. Although the NHS doesn't allow different wages, the reality looks often different. But in general the negative effects occur mainly in the lower controlled private sector (Buchan, 2004).

4 Strategies

According to the controversy of brain drain from African countries, the NHS implemented 1999 a guideline, which should avoid the immigration from people of South Africa and the Caribbean. But the number of immigrants increased nevertheless (Tab.3, Tab.4). The private sector and professional organizations often aren't a part of this agreement and furthermore many other countries suffer from brain drain and there no solutions were found so far. Different Codes of Practice for nurses' migration are existing worldwide. They claim fostering high standards in recruitment and the need of agreement from the donor government to the migration. But a final solution for the negative effect hasn't been found so far (Aiken, 2004; Buchan, 2002; Kline, 2003; Stilwell, 2004).

Country	1998/ 1999	1999/ 2000	2000/ 2001	2001/ 2002	% change 1998/99 to 1999/2000	% change 1999/2000 to 2000/01	% change 2000/ 01 to 2001/02
South Africa	599	1,460	1,086	2,114	+144	-25	+95
Caribbean	221	425	261	248	+92	-39	-5
Zimbabwe	52	221	382	473	+325	+73	+24
Ghana	40	74	140	195	+85	+89	+39
India	30	96	289	994	+220	+201	+244
Nigeria	179	208	347	432	+16	+67	+25
Philippines	52	1,052	3,396	7235	+1,923	+223	+113
(Total non-EU registrants)	(3,621)	(5,988)	(8403)	(13,721)	(+65)	(+40)	(+63)

Tab.3: Impact of 1999 ethical recruitment guidelines- registrants from selected countries. Before and after implementation of the guidelines in November 1999 (Buchan, 2002, p.18)

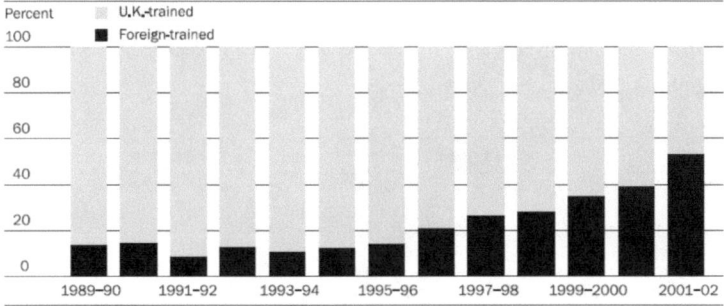

SOURCE: J. Buchan et al., *International Nurse Mobility: Trends and Policy Implications* (Geneva: World Health Organization, 2003).
NOTES: UKCC is the United Kingdom Central Council for Nursing, Midwifery, and Health Visiting. NMC is the Nursing Midwifery Council.

Tab. 4: Percentage Of New U.K.-Trained And Foreign-Trained Nurses Added To The UKCC/NMC Register, 1989-90 to 2001-02Aiken, 2004, p.73)

Conclusion

Migration is not negative in general- in contrast both sides can benefit from each other. But different points need to be addressed in the future to work on the negative effects of migration:

To bring all solutions on a evidential and valid bases, more data about nurses' migration is necessary. Lack of data is a basic problem, which needs to be addressed by regular exchange of current data between the countries to understand the problem more and to avoid poor solutions due to wrong assumptions (Stilwell, 2004).

Donor countries should work on minimizing the push- factors. Those, who go due to educational factors, could be held back by higher education, higher wages, team-work or supervision. Not everything will be possible, but targeted incentives will probably reduce the number of emigrating nurses and increase the situation for donor countries in two ways: retention of nurses and higher standard through incentives (Stilwell, 2004).

The only long- term and real successful strategy seems to be a higher investment of destination-countries in their own nursing resources to minimize the dependency on oversea nurses and from countries with nurse shortages. If not, the current -and in the future even more extreme- migration to the UK is not controllable and thereby negative effects are implicated (Aiken, 2004; Kline, 2004; Stilwell, 2004; Buchan, 2002).

Literature

Aiken, L.H., Buchan, J., Sochalski, J., Nichols, B., Powell, M. (2004) Trends In International Migration. *Health Affairs* [online], 23 (3). pp.73-77. Available online: http://content.healthaffairs.org/cgi/content/full/23/3/69?hits=10&FIRSTINDEX=0 &AUTHOR1=Barbara%2BNichols&ck=nck&SEARCHID=1&gca=healthaff%3 B23%2F3%2F69& [active: June, the 4ᵗʰ. 2010].

Buchan, J. (2002) *International recruitment of nurses: United Kingdom case study* [online]. Edingburgh, Queen Margaret University College. Available online: https://www.rcn.org.uk/__data/assets/pdf_file/0010/78544/001814.pdf [active: June, the 4ᵗʰ 2010].

Kline, D.S. (2003) Push and Pull Factors in International Nurse Migration. *Journal of Nursing Scholarship* [online]. 35 (2), pp. 107-111. Available online: http://www3.interscience.wiley.com/cgi-bin/fulltext/118855563/PDFSTART [active: June, the 4ᵗʰ 2010].

Stilwell, B., Diallo, K., Zurn, P., Vujicic, M., Adams, O., Dal Poz, M. (2004) Migration of health-care workers from developing countries: strategic approaches to its management. *Bulletin of the World Health Organization* [online]. 82 (8), pp.595-599. Available online: http://www.scielosp.org/scielo.php?pid=S0042-96862004000800009&script=sci_arttext&tlng=en [active: June, the 4ᵗʰ 2010].